15 minute habits

LITTLE STEPS, BIG RESULTS.

Stress Less

HERRON

Hello

The power of habit. It is not to be underestimated. It is both *how* we live our lives, and *what* happens to us.

But the good news is that success lies in the little things – routines, reminders, behaviours, thoughts – that you can easily adopt (or drop).

With this interactive journal in hand, all you need to do is commit 15 minutes of your time, and the belief that you can make it happen.

You will find 50 ideas to choose from. Each one could take you further in the direction of your goal for less stress in your life. Try one, a few, or all of them, and then record your experiences in the reflection section at the back of the book.

Less stress – inner peace, acceptance and a sense that your life is 'just right'. However you define it, you can be it. This book will show you how.

Contents

INTRO

YOU ARE YOUR HABITS

It's perhaps an extreme way of putting it, but it contains a compelling truth: the repeated actions that you take every day play a big part in making you who you are. This book is about changing your life, 15 minutes at a time – even five minutes at a time – by using the power of habit.

FIRING AND WIRING

Our brains are plastic and can be moulded. Neuropsychologist Donald Hebb coined his famous phrase in 1949: 'Neurons that fire together wire together.' It means that when you repeat an activity regularly, the structure of your brain changes to make that activity easier and more automatic. To instil a habit, you simply have to do it – not once, but over and over again. In time it will become so automatic that you'll barely notice you're doing it.

IDENTITY-DRIVEN CHANGE

We are driven to change because our current reality doesn't suit our desired one. If you want to start doing breathing exercises or meditating it's because that suits the mental picture you want for yourself: *I am a peaceful and relaxed person.* Understand this fact, and you can reframe your desire for the new habit in a more positive and holistic way. The bigger picture will help you make the small changes required to gradually become that identity.

HOW TO USE THIS BOOK

The following pages will take you through tips and tricks for how to create positive change through the power of habit. It will give you a host of ideas for new habits to eliminate stress and attain inner peace – and how to embed them in your everyday. The habits are categorised into the big themes that matter to help you achieve your goal of less stress in your life. Pick something easy that resonates with you, and try to implement it. Experiment, review, reflect and reset – don't be afraid to play around with different ideas until you find something that sticks. Habits can be tricky to get off the ground – but once they're ingrained, they have the power to change your life.

> 'Practice isn't the thing you do once you're good. It's the thing you do that makes you good.'
>
> MALCOLM GLADWELL

HABIT-BUILDING TRICKS

START SMALL

Research tells us that willpower is like a muscle. Overuse can exhaust it. If you rely on motivation alone to power your new habits you'll hit struggletown before the end of the day. So trick your willpower by starting with an action so easy you don't need a lot of motivation to follow through. If you want to do a 30-minute yoga session each morning, start with a single two-minute pose. Rather than starting with 50 push-ups a day, start with five. Make the habit so tiny that you need almost zero motivation to do it.

JUST SHOW UP

From that humble base, build up gradually. Very gradually. Go slower than you think you need to. Don't exceed the power of your motivation. Focus on being consistent – regular repetition is how the habit will become embedded in your routine. Don't even think about reaching your goal – just focus on showing up.

SAY IT OUT LOUD

Don't underestimate the power of the spoken word. Stating your intention clearly and unequivocally makes it more real. Be sure to align your intention with the identity that's underpinning it – so, for example, if you're trying to cut a sugar habit and you're tempted by an offer of cake, say out loud, 'I don't eat sweets.'

DON'T THINK, DO

We can be fooled into thinking we've started a habit when actually we're just procrastinating. Say you want to start a creative habit. You buy some watercolour paints, then some nice paper to paint on. You follow some social media accounts for inspiration. Then you need to find some brushes, and a box to store all your new painting gear in ... Stop! Simply do. Start drawing with what's at hand, now, for five minutes a day – a pencil, a pen, a Sharpie – and gather better materials as you go. Gradually.

MAKE IT EASY

Friction is the enemy of forming habits. In the early stages, you need the habit to be as easy as possible. Remove barriers, let the new habit flow seamlessly into the current of your daily life. Think about how your life and routine is set up to either make it tricky to start your new habit, or easy to continue with habits you want to break. What could you change?

SEE IT, DO IT

One positive change is to adapt your environment to naturally encourage your new habit. Keep a jug of water on your desk, stop stocking your kitchen pantry with chocolate, keep your running shoes by the door or your yoga mat in plain sight in the living room. Use your surroundings to provide triggers and reinforce your behaviour.

HABIT STACKING

Piggyback your new desired habits onto ones that are already in your routine. Do an audit of your current habits – everything from your first morning cup of tea to brushing your teeth before you go to bed at night. List them, and identify where you might be able to seamlessly slot in a new habit, for example a five-minute stretching session before your morning shower, or a walk after dinner. Make your existing habits, already so strongly ingrained, act as cues to strengthen your new ones.

ONE BABY STEP

Nudge yourself into your habit by planting the seed and preparing the terrain. Take a small step that edges you closer to action – you'll create your own trigger so that the habit comes easier. For example, if you want to start gardening for 30 minutes a day, instead just get out your gardening gloves and tools and take them outside. That's all. Next time, maybe pull out a weed or two. No more. The power in this approach is that once you start, it's easier to continue – you may even find it hard to resist taking the next step.

THE ROLE OF REWARDS

Adding a reward is a powerful way to instil your new habit. It associates a pleasure with the new behaviour, motivating your brain to repeat the reward-winning action. Over time, the reward becomes less important as the habit becomes ingrained and its benefits become more obvious and intrinsically rewarding. You can use rewards as a kind of bribe to motivate the behaviour, perhaps simultaneously – for example, do your daily admin (desirable habit) at the same as drinking your morning coffee (pleasurable reward). Or, allow yourself to do something you enjoy afterwards – for example, after going for a run, relax and scroll your socials for 10 minutes or read a chapter of your book.

REVIEW AND RESET

The only downside of good habits is that when they become part of your routine they can get stale. You put them on autopilot and forget to fine-tune, adapt and improve. Avoid this by doing an annual review and asking yourself what you've learned, what's changed in your life, and how you can take things to the next level, or whether maybe it's time to seek out something new.

> 'Every action you take is a vote for the type of person you wish to become.'
>
> JAMES CLEAR

HONOURING YOUR COMMITMENTS TO YOURSELF

STAY THE COURSE

Hang in there. Habits take time to make stick (estimates range from 59 to 90 days). Be patient and be kind to yourself. Stay connected to your purpose. For some, motivation is jogged by tracking numbers and ticking boxes. That's great if it works for you, but also remember the bigger picture of what you are doing and why. Repetition and practise can be boring – but they're worth it.

BACK ON THE BIKE

You'll fall off from time to time, and you'll face challenges to your resolve. Don't be discouraged by these bumps in the road. Cling to (true) clichés like 'Practise makes perfect' and 'Nothing easy is worth doing'. Try to learn from your mistakes and stay focused on the sense of accomplishment that comes from continuing to achieve in this aspect of your life.

BE YOUR OWN COACH

Another helpful cliché: 'Be a coach, not a critic'. Don't beat yourself up with negative self-talk if you don't hit your goals (that never helped anyone improve), but do hold yourself accountable. Create a penalty for failing to do your habit: maybe it's a donation to charity, or you give up the right to Netflix or socials for an evening. Whatever feels like it will be the most motivating.

FIND YOUR TRIBE

Mutual motivation is a powerful thing. It's much easier to stick to things when we're in a group. Surround yourself with people in pursuit of the same goals as you – join a bootcamp crew, a crafting circle, a casual running team, a writers' group – whatever your proposed new habit, think about how you can find other people to reinforce and enrich it. Even if your tribe is a virtual one, the benefits will be enormous.

SECTION ONE

Setting up for success

B

Today is going to be a beautiful day

IT'S THE LITTLE THINGS

Five minutes here and there might not seem like much. But it's often the small details in life that bring us the most joy and smooth the path to a less stressful life. By taking our focus off the big goals and instead taking a micro approach to positive change, we give ourselves the benefit of small, sweet successes. Take a sense of accomplishment from each small step along the way, and feel the positive feedback of a job (gradually) well done.

TAKE CONTROL

You have the power to shape your day – and by extension, your world. The small tweaks you make to enhance your life build up step by step to a transformed, peaceful you, free of stress and angst. Believe in the process, have faith in yourself and keep putting one foot in front of the other. Control what you can, and let the rest follow.

BELIEVE IT, BE IT

Don't buy in to negative hype. When you're trying to make real change, a little blind faith goes a long way. The outcome depends on only one thing – your mindset. When the inevitable doubts arise and threaten your resolve, do your best to calm them and simply *do*. Action is the best way to quieten down a sceptical inner voice. Believe it: *I am peaceful*. And be it.

M

Move your body

SHAKE IT

Trying to integrate more exercise into your life? You're in good company – most people say they'd like to do more physical activity. And for good reason. Being active is not only vital to keeping weight under control, it strengthens bones and muscles, improves heart health and boosts energy. It makes you a healthy human.

OILING THE MACHINE

And there's more beyond the headline benefits. Exercise is essential for a happy endocrine system, and it regulates levels of adrenaline and cortisol, the body's stress hormones. Plus, it boosts the production of endorphins, the brain's feel-good neurotransmitters, our natural painkillers and mood elevators.

HAPPY SIDE-EFFECTS

All those physical benefits mean great outcomes for your sense of inner peace. Good news for troubled slumber: physical activity makes it easier to drift off and improves sleep quality. It has also been shown to reduce stress and depression, sharpen focus and help calm a busy mind. Physical wellbeing and mental wellbeing are two sides of the same shiny coin.

BODY HEALTH HABITS

They call sitting the new smoking. Sedentary lifestyles are largely to blame for our movement deficit. Simply standing up is a starting point – get into the habit of standing and stretching and soon it becomes essential. Seize opportunities to move – walk around when you're on the phone, stand up on public transport, invest in a standing desk. Movement begets movement – the more you move, the more you'll feel like moving. It's a truly virtuous circle.

SD

Slow down some

FAST-LANE LIFE

We live in a culture of busy-ness. If you're not in a rush, you're somehow not doing enough. We complain about how full our schedules are – so many appointments, too much work, endless commitments – with a tinge of boastfulness. To be run off one's feet is to be in demand; to be busy is to be achieving.

PRESS PAUSE

And for many of us, juggling family, work, friends and life projects, time is precious and too scarce. That's what makes it even more important to be aware of the need to slow down every once in a while. Awareness is the first step – become conscious of the fact that inner peace is not something we can find in the midst of stress.

STOP, BREATHE, BE

In this book you'll find the power of breath mentioned more than once. It's a simple switch we can flick that reminds us to pause for a moment and be still. Shift your focus and linger in a nourishing moment of peace. Becoming aware that this oasis exists inside you and can be called on when you need it is a gift that can sustain you through the trickiest moments.

TAKE A TIME OUT

And it's in those tricky moments that it's vital to give yourself permission to pause. You are your own time-keeper. When you need time to process, reflect and choose, know that you have the right to slow things down and start a habit of doing so.

SAVOUR LIFE

The endless rush can mean that we forget to simply appreciate. Mindfulness is about being in the moment so we can open our eyes – and all our senses – to all that is around us. Slowing down makes life better enabling us to manage stress and learn little tricks to help you invite peace in.

RES

Respect yourself and your environment

SET YOUR BOUNDARIES

Finding moments of peace, slowing down and listening to yourself will make your own values ever clearer to you. Ask yourself whether you're living by them. That makes it easier to identify and avoid what's toxic, what doesn't serve you, what you need to let go of. Honour your needs. Seek out what makes you feel good, nourished, respected; say 'no' to the rest.

MOULD YOUR SURROUNDINGS

There's a sense of creation in making your life what you want it to be, and you'll find that spills over into the spaces you inhabit. As the setting for many of your habits, your home plays an important role – use it to reinforce the actions you want to take, and make sure it reflects the identity that you desire for yourself. Your sense of inner peace should be mirrored in the spaces where you spend the most time.

RB

Relax that body of yours

CHOOSE YOUR METHOD

You can use your body as the means to help you combat stress and instil a sense of inner peace. Physical relaxation is a road to the calm, serene self that you seek, and you can travel it on a variety of vehicles: meditation, yoga, body scanning, vagus nerve stimulation, massage (by yourself or others), acupressure ... Try them all. Choose your favourite and make it a habit.

STRETCH AND SOOTHE

The benefits of a regular yoga practice – for both body and mind – are well documented, and a worthy aim. But you don't need to make a heavy commitment to do an hour of yoga a day. A few targeted stretches will do you a world of good, especially if you spend lots of time behind a desk. Morning stretches, before-bed stretches or once-an-hour one-minute stretch breaks – start a stretch habit to tap into life's most readily available anti-stress therapy.

PEACE HACKS

There are other ways you can get a relaxation quick fix. The vagus nerve – the body's communication superhighway, running from your brain to your gut – plays a big role in regulating the parasympathetic nervous system, which has a calming influence in your day-to-day. A little vagus stimulation – easily accessible by singing, gargling or a cold-water face splash – can give you a sense of peaceful wellbeing. You'll find tricks like this in the pages that follow to help you chill out and calm down.

EY

Express your amazing self

FIRST, LISTEN

Einstein said it best: 'Curiosity is more important than knowledge.' Be endlessly curious, especially when it comes to yourself. Question yourself and your motivations – not to second-guess them, but to seek new insight and understanding. Always wonder why and how, look under the surface. Self-exploration leads to greater self-awareness, which will help you find the best paths out of stress and towards inner peace.

LET IT FLOW

Journalling can help. Whether you let your inner thoughts run free in a stream-of-consciousness mind dump, journal your gratitude or simply write down your experiences as you take this journey of self-transformation, expressing yourself in words will give you greater clarity and insight.

FEEL THE FLOW

The act of creation is a way to activate a deeply calming state of flow. Whether you're working in the garden, doodling, playing an instrument or crafting a mosaic masterpiece, when you create your mind is fully in the present moment – the only place you'll find peace. Starting a new hobby (which is a special kind of habit, but a habit nonetheless) is a way of marking out this intention to spend regular time in a blissful flow state.

S

Simplify your life

CLEAR THE CLUTTER

Make space for tranquillity. Think of your environment as a mirror for your internal state – you can't quieten mental noise when you're surrounded by physical clutter. So tidy, reduce, donate – get rid of everything that doesn't contribute to your life in some way – and feel the calming effect on your state of mind. Re-organise your space with your new habits in mind, so that your environment provides cues and reinforces your desired behaviours. Take control of your environment and you're on the way to taking control of your daily routines and your state of mind.

REDUCE THE NOISE

But it's not just your home environment that might need a clean-out. Turn down the volume so you can better hear yourself think. Declutter your schedule to find time to slow down. Rethink your technology habits to free your consciousness to reflect and create. Let go of unhelpful thought patterns and ruminations. Maybe you even need to examine certain relationships in your life that aren't good for you. Simplifying is about focusing on – and spending your time with – the things that nourish your inner self.

NR

Create nourishing routines

THE POWER OF REPETITION

By definition, a habit is an action you repeat over and over again, generally every day. Embedding positive habits into your daily routines is critical to their success, and in this book you'll find tips on how to do that. One way is to incorporate new habits into your existing routines, already so ingrained in your day-to-day life. Use them as cues and add new steps to help combat stress and deliver you nourishment and inner peace instead.

DAILY RITUALS

Your morning and evening routines are probably so well set that you don't even think about them. They're fertile ground for inserting new, positive habits. Adding a new step – making your bed or scraping your tongue – is as easy as slipping it into the flow of the routine. Other routines may be less obvious – for example, transition routines that take you from one state to another, such as your getting-home-from-work routine. Think about a mindful habit you could add to make this ritual more nourishing.

GOOD TRIGGERS

Your habitual everyday actions can be repurposed as positive triggers to spark nourishing new habits. Experiment – try different triggers, different times of day. You may find that taking a moment to connect with spirit works better for you in the morning – make it a habit to take five minutes to breathe and connect after you drink your morning cuppa. To remind yourself to drink plenty of water, set your water bottle on your desk for the next day as part of your after-dinner clean-up. Tiny tweaks can have big results.

C

Connect with yourself and others

YOUR PEACEFUL PLACE

Use the power of habit to strengthen your relationship with yourself. A regular return to your centre – the place where you are truly at peace – will improve your self-awareness and nourish your soul. Making it a habit to check in with yourself – whether at times of stress or on a daily basis as part of a mindfulness or breathing practice – has wide-ranging benefits. Connect with your breath, your senses, your spirit. The more connected you are to yourself, the stronger connections you can make with others.

BE PRESENT

We spend so much time multi-tasking and scheduled to the hilt that we can overlook the importance of slowing down to take real time with the important people in our lives. Habit can help us remember. Dedicating small but meaningful moments in the day to be present with others nourishes relationships and strengthens bonds. Be intentional and let others know how much they mean to you. Reach out, make the first move, surprise and delight loved ones with unexpected gestures. Let them feel that you embrace and accept them as they are, without trying to change them.

G

Give back

CALCULATED KINDNESS

It may seem like an oxymoron, but there's nothing wrong with being intentional about acts of kindness. Creating a kindness habit will gradually rewire your mind, making spontaneous acts of kindness come more naturally. Start by doing one small good thing for someone each day, and watch as the feel-good effects come back to you, in ways that you may not expect.

GIVING IS GREAT

Explore ways that you can create a habit that helps you give something back. Donations don't have to be about money. You can donate time, expertise or care. Being of service connects you with your wider community and humanity as a whole; dedicating time to help others will teach you patience, kindness and resilience. You'll feel a greater sense of purpose and belonging, a deeper sense of inner peace, all of which will help minimise stress.

FEEL-GOOD VIBES

When you're acting for the benefit of someone else, you're taking the focus off yourself and your own problems. This simple shift of attention can lighten the load of worry and rumination. Plus, knowing you've done something good for someone is sure to bring a smile to your lips (thanks to that endorphin rush you just triggered). Making others happy with no expectation of reward or recompense makes the world a better place – that's a good habit to get into.

SECTION TWO

Stress less habits

CONTENTS OF HABITS

01

MORNING PAGES

15 MINUTES

A daily nudge for the creative spirit within, this writing habit – three A4 pages of longhand, stream-of-consciousness prose first thing in the morning – was invented by creativity guru Julia Cameron in the 1990s. Designed to kick-start the stalled pens of blocked writers, this daily date with your inner voice is a powerful habit for wannabe novelists and a hotline to your authentic self.

DO THIS

1. Source a cute journal and keep it at your bedside.
2. Write the pages the moment you awaken, before getting up.
3. Morning pages are for your eyes only – keep them private.

'Each morning, as we face the page, we meet ourselves.'

JULIA CAMERON

EY C

I write.

02
SET YOUR ALARM

30 SECONDS

Start your day as you mean to go on – by taking control of your time. This simple habit puts the day's first decision in your hands, giving you pole position to make the most of those all-important first couple of hours.

Be mindful of setting the mood when you set the alarm – choose your favourite banger for a high-energy start, or ambient sounds to ease you into wakefulness. Whatever works for you. Avoid hitting snooze (it'll just make you feel more tired) and slide straight into your morning routine.

'Each morning we are born again. What we do today is what matters most.'

JACK KORNFIELD

B NR

I start every day positively.

03

STRETCH

5 MINUTES

Whether it's to ease into your day, as an afternoon recharge or an evening wind-down, a stretch a day has serious long-term benefits.

Of all the physical exercise you can do, stretching is perhaps the most precious one to make a habit of. With regular practice, it will help increase the range of motion in your joints, improve blood circulation and posture and alleviate muscular tension throughout your body.

As well as all that, stretching reduces stress and releases tension. It's a great way to give yourself a mental break, to revitalise energy and calm the mind.

To get all this good stuff, you don't need to commit to an hour-long yoga class. A simple 5-minute stretching session is all you need to raise your body – and mood – to a higher plane.

M

I take care of my body.

DO THIS

1. Child's pose: On all fours, reach your arms forward, sit back on your heels and rest your forehead on the floor.

2. Cat/cow: On all fours, arch and then round your back as you inhale and exhale.

3. Shoulder stretches: Lace your fingers together and raise your arms above your head.

4. Forward bend: Fold at your hips, keeping your torso long and your knees slightly bent, hands reaching for the floor.

5. Neck rotations: Slowly rotate your head in a circle, clockwise then anticlockwise.

DID YOU KNOW?

Our joints can lose up to 50% of their range of motion as we age.

04

COOL AND CLEANSE

5 MINUTES

Meet your vagus nerve. It's one of the cranial nerves connecting brain to body and has a major role in how both function. As the primary nerve of the parasympathetic nervous system – that's the zen counterbalance to the sympathetic nervous system responsible for the 'fight or flight' response – it acts as a stress neutraliser. Stimulating it triggers your body to relax.

Your vagus nerve is connected to your vocal cords and the muscles at the back of your throat. When you sing or hum in the shower, you stimulate the vagus and call on your body's natural ability to feel good – so if you don't it's time to start! Gargling has the same effect, intensified.

While you're in the bathroom, chill out. Cold showers are thought to improve the metabolism, build the immune system and be an effective pain-fighter. Not only that, a rush of cold can have a positive impact on psychological strength – slightly uncomfortable activities like this build willpower and the neural pathways that contribute to resilience.

RB NR

I know how to make myself feel good.

DO THIS

1. Gargle loudly for up to 30 seconds after brushing your teeth morning and night.
2. Turn on the cold tap – start with 30 seconds at the start or end of your normal shower, and gradually build up to 2 minutes.
3. Sing or hum in the shower – the louder the better.
4. Immerse your forehead, eyes and at least two-thirds of both cheeks into cold water to stimulate your vagus nerve.

DID YOU KNOW?

The vagus is a communication bridge between brain and gut – it's why we experience 'gut feelings'.

05

SAY GOODBYE WITH CARE

5 MINUTES

Mornings can be a mad rush. And that's exactly why a moment of care and love before 9 am carries extra weight. Before you run out the door (or lock yourself away in your office), take a meaningful moment to farewell your loved ones(s). A kiss, a hug, some thoughtful words – make it considered and heartfelt. Listen, be present and place your focus completely on them, resisting the temptation to be carried forward into your day. It will add a glow to your morning as much as it does theirs.

DO THIS

1. Leave a note telling your loved one you'll miss them during the day.
2. Follow up with a text – even if it's just some kiss emojis.
3. Don't forget your pets!

'This is not a goodbye, my darling, this is a thank you.'

NICHOLAS SPARKS

SD C G

I make my loved ones feel special.

06
MAKE YOUR BED

5 MINUTES

It's partly basic hygiene. Your bed is home to countless dust mites (yes, sorry), and making your bed exposes them to clean air, causing them to dry up and perish.

But making your bed is also a statement of positive intent for the day, the launching pad for the good habits that follow. It sets the scene for how you want the rest of your day to unfold – uncluttered, neat and mindful. And it's a simple gesture of self-care – as you shake out that doona and fluff up those pillows, you prepare your nest for the restful night's sleep to come.

DID YOU KNOW?

People who make their beds are 19% more likely to get a good night's sleep than those who don't.

RES NR

My home is well-ordered and comfortable.

07

LEAVE THE HOUSE MINDFULLY

5 MINUTES

Do you consistently rush out in a state of semi-panic, sure that you've forgotten something and anxious that you've left the oven on or the cat locked in? Smooth your morning routine by getting into the habit of leaving home with purpose.

Set the scene by making sure that your environment is organised efficiently. Do you have a regular place to put your keys, hang your bag, store all those everyday going-out items (sunglasses, umbrella, charger ...)? Keep them all together if you can, close to the front door.

Write a list of all those tiny morning tasks: do breakfast dishes, feed dog, close bathroom window ... Whatever they are, write them down and put the note on the fridge door. Before you step out the front door, pause for one moment to mentally check off that list.

And then walk out, closing the door behind you with total peace of mind.

SD RES

I am efficient and well-organised.

08

FOCUS ON THE BREATH

5 MINUTES

A few deep, mindful breaths is the quickest, easiest pick-me-up we can access. Yet how often do we get to the end of the day and realise that we haven't really filled our lungs once?

Getting into a breathing habit gives you the opportunity to stimulate your vagus nerve and tap into some natural stress relief, as well as slowing things down for a calming bubble of centred, grounded time in your day.

Choose a moment that makes sense for you – it can be anytime, anywhere. While you're waiting for the kettle to boil, under the shower, during your commute, at the start of your morning tea break – choose a trigger that is already part of your daily routine. Find a simple breathing exercise you can slip into, and add a check-in moment at the end to connect with yourself. It will be the most well-spent five minutes of your day.

SD RB

DID YOU KNOW?

Breathing is the only autonomous system of the body that we can also control.

I am calm and peaceful.

09
TECH CONTROL HABIT

5 MINUTES

S SD RES

I have a healthy relationship with technology.

Social media, streaming platforms, instant messaging – there's no doubt technology is an incredible enabler of communication, learning and entertainment. But it's boundless, and unless we form healthy habits it can do more harm than good.

Platforms operate by commanding your attention, and do everything they can to keep it. Wrest back control by deciding exactly how much of your day you want to spend on TikTok or answering emails or binge-watching series.

Remember: it's up to you which applications you install on your phone and if you set notifications for each one. You can even set limits on the time you spend on individual apps in your phone's settings. Use tech to help yourself set healthy tech habits.

DO THIS

1. Turn off messaging, social media and email notifications.
2. Check messages and email four times daily only: 9 am, noon, 3 pm and 6 pm.
3. Set a block of technology-free time each day.
4. Make mealtimes screen free.

10

DO THE LIFE ADMIN

5 MINUTES

Think of it as oiling the wheels of your existence. Health appointments, paying bills, tax returns ... Individually they're not a big time drag, but they punch above their weight in stressfulness when they start to build up.

Banish the 'Have I forgotten something important?' blues by building a habit around your life admin. Start with a list – paper, Excel, Notion, whatever works for you. When a life admin thing pops up, add it automatically to your list.

Decide on a timeslot – maybe it's your Monday morning teatime task, or your wind-down Wednesday afternoon. Make it weekly and book it in. That's your life admin slot when you'll deal with all these little tasks. Simply building an easy, reliable system will help your life hum like a well-oiled machine.

'The point is to master the habit of showing up.'

JAMES CLEAR

S

My life is in order.

11

BODY SCAN

5 MINUTES

Taking a moment out of the day to slow down and listen to your body helps raise self-awareness – mental, emotional and physical. This quick, nurturing meditation is a great after-work grounding exercise, and particularly effective as a pre-sleep wind-down.

DO THIS

1. Lie down, close your eyes and take a few deep breaths.
2. Bring your awareness to your feet. Observe any sensations without judgement.
3. Move your attention upwards, slowly scanning your entire body. Notice any tension, pain or pressure.
4. If your attention wanders, gently direct it back until you finish at the crown of your head.

SD RB C

I am in touch with my body.

'Awareness is like the sun. When it shines on things, they are transformed.'

THICH NHAT HANH

12

TAP INTO FEELINGS OF DISCOMFORT

10 MINUTES

Feeling awkward can be a signal that there's something deeper going on. We can find ourselves in a situation that makes us feel uncomfortable without really knowing why. Maybe you're in a harmless conversation that suddenly becomes confronting, or plans change and leave you outlandishly disappointed.

Get into the habit of investigating an out-of-context reaction to explore what's underneath. Instead of letting the feeling linger and morph into full-blown anxiety, linger for a moment. Delve in. Take the chance to learn more about yourself, your fears and your deepest beliefs. It might be the opportunity for a breakthrough.

DO THIS

1. When you feel discomfort, remind yourself not to take it at face value.
2. Remove yourself from the situation if you need to.
3. Turn towards your emotions with acceptance.
4. Try to identify the emotion: is it anger, fear, sadness?
5. Inquire gently, what made me feel this way?

EY C

I am very self-aware.

13

EAT MINDFULLY

1 HOUR

SD NR

I have a healthy relationship with food.

Too often, we multi-task our meals. We dine watching a screen, lunch while working, grab a bite on the run from one appointment to the next. It's not good for our digestion or our state of mind.

Mindful eating regards the meal as a meditation. It's a chance to pause, pay attention and engage the senses, noting the colours, smells, tastes and textures of the food and how it makes you feel.

Mark mealtimes by changing your environment. Avoid eating on the couch – sit at a table, use a place-mat, light a candle. Pour sparkling water into a nice glass. Create a sense that this is a special moment of the day, when other things are put aside.

Take a moment to honour the food before you eat, gratefully acknowledging the ingredients and how they arrived to your table. Take small bites, chewing thoroughly. Slowing down helps you stop when you've had enough – the body's signals to the brain to tell you you're full can take 15 to 20 minutes to kick in.

Getting into the habit of mindful eating is key to having a healthy relationship with food. And research has shown that it improves digestion, regulates the appetite and helps us enjoy our food much more.

DO THIS

1. Eat at around the same time each day, and don't skip meals.
2. Respect your lunch hour. Don't eat 'al desko' – enjoy the meal with others, outside or in the lunch room.
3. Chew each mouthful until you can taste the essence of the food.
4. Pause periodically to pay attention to the sensations you're experiencing.
5. Stop when you're 80% full.
6. Eat plant-based and non-processed food that nourishes your body, and prioritise your gut health.
7. If you have time, go for a 15-minute walk after your meal.

DID YOU KNOW?

Over 90% of the digestion and absorption of nutrients takes place in the small intestine, not the stomach.

14

BE PRESENT WITH OTHERS

5 MINUTES

SD C G

I make meaningful connections with other people.

Like everything else in life, peace feels even better when shared. It can be as simple as being present and acknowledging the beauty of a moment with a person dear to you. Share a mindful cup of tea and a peaceful moment with a friend or loved one.

DO THIS

1. Pause: Take a few moments to sit with your cup of tea before you start drinking it.
2. Relax: Breathe and be still in the shared comfortable silence.
3. Enjoy: Sip the tea, savour its warming spread and sensual aroma. Smile at each other with appreciation of this simple moment.

> 'While there is tea, there is hope.'
>
> ARTHUR WING PINERO

15

STAY REGULATED

5 MINUTES

NR C

I am emotionally well balanced.

Emotional ups and downs are normal. We feel frustrated when we're stuck in traffic. We feel sad when we miss our loved ones. We might get angry if someone lets us down. But our emotions can veer off-track. We might over-invest emotional energy in a situation that doesn't require it, and find it difficult to evaluate clearly.

That's when the habit of self-regulation comes into play. It's all about pausing between feeling and reaction. It encourages us to slow down for a bit and act after objectively evaluating the situation. That allows us to scale back if necessary, so our level of intensity more appropriately matches the situation. Learn your emotional cues so you know when to hit the pause button.

DO THIS

1. Take a few deep breaths.
2. Change your environment: go outside or take a quick walk.
3. Connect with your senses: name five things you can see, hear, smell, feel and taste.
4. Repeat a positive affirmation, like: 'I am not my feelings' or 'I am allowed to feel this way'.

16

SAY NO

5 MINUTES

Knowing – and honouring – your boundaries is a superpower. You don't have to act on every idea your boss comes up with, or join all of your friends' plans, or take on all the responsibilities for your family life.

One of the best things you can do for your mental health is to learn to say no when you are tired, too busy, or asked to do something that you simply don't want to do.

Don't feel guilty. Just say no. After the first time, once you get into the habit, it will get easier and easier.

'When you say "yes" to others, make sure you are not saying "no" to yourself.'

PAULO COELHO

RES

I always act in line with my values.

17
REHYDRATE

5 MINUTES

We all know the importance of keeping hydrated. It's just a matter of remembering to do it. Positive triggers are your friends: when you see the water, you'll drink the water. Two litres a day is an easy habit to keep when you're surrounded by the stuff.

Be mindful of drinks that can dehydrate you – coffee, tea, alcohol – they're not a one-for-one replacement for H2O. If water bores you, add a touch of excitement with lemon slices, mint leaves or cucumber chunks. Herbal teas and tisanes are your wintertime hydration superpower. And always avoid sugary drinks.

DO THIS

1. Keep a reusable water bottle in your bag so you're never without it.
2. Have a jug of water sitting on your desk as you work.
3. Make a big jug of iced tea every morning and keep it in the fridge.

RES NR

I drink enough water.

18

MAKE TIME TO BE OUTSIDE

15 MINUTES

How often have you arrived at the end of a day and realised that you haven't ventured outside once? Our lifestyles mean that we spend great chunks of time indoors, often in front of a screen, so it's important to mindfully build time into the day for sun, fresh air and the feeling of freedom.

Spending time in nature is linked to a host of benefits: improved attention, lower stress, better sleep, even upticks in empathy and cooperation. Green spaces act as a balm for busy brains, restoring our ability to pay attention and making us feel more positive.

Even if you can't step outside your front door into a wild forest, you have access to sky, sun and stars – plus, part of the benefit of being outdoors is a chance to change your frame, stretch your legs, breathe deeply and pay attention.

Make a date with the outdoors part of your daily routine by deciding on the best trigger. A quick turn around the block before you start work, eating lunch outside, a walk the park before or after dinner – make your cue a daily habit you already follow.

NR C

I get fresh air and sunshine every day.

DO THIS

1. Sit in silence and soak up the warmth of some rays.
2. Lie down under a tree and look up at the clouds.
3. Take a mindful walk: open your senses and observe 10 things.
4. Take your shoes off and stand or walk on the grass or sand.
5. Find your favourite local tree and visit it every day to say hello.
6. Stargaze.

DID YOU KNOW?

Vitamin D from sunlight helps the body produce melatonin, a hormone that supports sleep.

19

CONNECT WITH SPIRIT

5 MINUTES

SD NR C

I am a spiritual person.

In the rush of daily life, the spiritual can be sideswiped by the urgency of the physical here-and-now. But this persistent sense of urgency contributes to stress. It's so important for our sense of inner peace to regularly take our focus within and connect with what's deeper inside us.

A few minutes a day is enough to pause and connect. Use props or cues to help you create a ritual – a crystal, tarot cards, a dedicated place in your home – and place your hand on your heart to centre. Imagine your thoughts going up to the Universe and returning with a loving, peaceful energy.

DO THIS

1. Find a comfortable position, or a favourite yoga pose.
2. Close your eyes.
3. Breathe deeply.

'When you make peace with yourself, you make peace with the world.'

MAHA GHOSANANDA

20

TAKE NO SIDES

5 MINUTES

It can seem as though the whole world has fallen into the habit of black-and-white thinking. It's the cause of so much conflict, from the global scale to the personal – this belief that there is one correct answer to everything (and I have that answer, so you must be wrong).

The proof is all around us that it's a dangerous habit to fall into. Guard against it. Even if you disagree with a person or an idea, you can coexist with them peacefully. Recognise when you are drawn to take sides in an argument, or judge another person, and find a way to disengage from that behaviour.

DO THIS

1. Avoid entering a debate you don't want to take sides in.
2. Present an alternative point of view without being attached to it.
3. Always keep the tone reasonable, light and non-personal.
4. If things get heated, change the subject completely or suggest you all do something different together.

EY C

I am non-judgemental.

21
SWAY AWAY

5 MINUTES

There's a reason why we rock babies in a cradle and why the rocking chair is a symbol of comfort and cosiness, idyllically enjoyed by grey-haired folk in country cottages. That gentle, rhythmic motion soothes the joints, stimulates the sense of balance and calms the nerves.

The vestibular system, located in the inner ear, helps us sense our physical position and supports our sense of balance and equilibrium. Swaying stimulates it. Vestibular stimulation is recognised as a powerful tool for self-soothing and it's a fast-track to centring and finding a moment of calm.

Make it a habit to sway for a moment at your stand-up desk or as you wait in line. Like a reed in the breeze, feel yourself move in rhythm with the world.

DO THIS

1. Stand with feet apart and knees slightly bent. Shift your weight slowly from side to side.
2. Consciously, slowly breathe through the nose in sync with the sway.
3. Want more? Consider joining a tai chi class.

M SD

I am balanced and strong.

22

FIND DAILY JOY

5 MINUTES

The potential for joy is all around us – it's just a matter of being in the right frame of mind to see it. Cultivating an attitude of positive observation – that is, being awake to the possibility of finding joy in the little things – is a habit of mind that helps keep your mood uplifted and your stress levels in check.

When a little something brings a smile to your lips or warmth to your heart, take note of what it was. You patted a dog? You said hello to a stranger in the street? You gave yourself a spritz in the perfume aisle? Remember it, keep it in mind and do it more often. Life is a series of moments – and the more joyful you make those tiny moments, the more joyful you make your life.

> 'Happiness often sneaks in through a door you didn't know you left open.'
>
> JOHN BARRYMORE

B SD NR

I am a happy person.

23

YOUR HEALTHY HOME HABITS

15 MINUTES

RES S NR

My home is a haven.

A messy and cluttered living environment can take a toll on your mood and motivation. And the more cleaning there is to do, the less you want to do it. By establishing some simple daily habits, you can stay on top of the chaos so that cleaning takes half the time. Plus, you get to live in a naturally healthy, simple and uncluttered home.

Put some thought into how your space is organised. Does everything have its dedicated spot in a logical, natural location? A basket or box on your desk for mail and papers; a dedicated charging station for devices; a bowl near the front door to collect keys, change and sunglasses. Make especially sure that your most-often misplaced items have their own home base.

When everything has its place, it's easier to get into the habit of putting things away as you use them. Every evening, spend 10 minutes cleaning up before you go to bed. A quick wipe-down and tidy-up as part of your bedtime routine means you'll always have the pleasure of waking up to an ordered home – it will reinforce the habit of keeping it tidy the next morning.

DO THIS

1. Have a place for shoes by the door and take them off when you enter.

2. Tidy your bathroom before you leave for work in the morning.

3. Wash the dishes after dinner – make it a mindful moment by listening to music or doing a guided meditation.

4. Burn a scented candle or diffuse essential oils during your night-time tidy-up to reinforce its calming effect.

5. Follow the one-in, one-out rule: when you acquire something new, donate something you already have.

'We should be choosing what we want to keep, not what we want to get rid of.'

MARIE KONDO

24

POWER OF PAUSE

1 MINUTE

SD EY

I am measured and considered in my responses.

The true power of the pause is knowing that it's always available. In our go-go-go culture we all feel under pressure to give the fast response, make the quick decision, move on to the next challenge without hesitation. But you are the keeper of the clock: it's your decision how fast, or slow, you want to take things.

Get into the habit of pausing before you respond. Imagine a giant pause button in your head. When a moment arrives that you're not sure what to do with, press that button. Take a beat or two to digest, consider, reset.

If you need to, shift your attention. Turn to look out the window. Close your eyes for a moment. Push back on the pressure for immediate reactions. It might feel strange at first, but those around will perceive you as thoughtful and measured – asserting control of taking a step back is most likely to gain their respect.

Remember, making progress isn't about doing everything – it's about doing the *right* things. Grant yourself the power to pause so you can see more clearly which those are.

DO THIS

1. When taking a momentary pause, take one deep breath. Follow it all the way in, all the way out.

2. If a moment is not enough, feel empowered to say, 'I need to think about that, I'll get back to you.'

3. Disengage if necessary – make a simple excuse and leave the room.

4. When you need to calm down, breathe in the 4–7–8 pattern for 2 minutes.

5. Recite a mantra to calm the spirit: 'With every breath, I feel more peaceful.'

DID YOU KNOW?

It's estimated that we each make upward of 35,000 decisions every day.

25

PRACTISE SELF-AWARENESS

5 MINUTES

SD EY C

I know myself well.

Research has shown that people who are more self-aware have higher self-esteem, achieve more and are better at creating and maintaining relationships. Being self-aware means observing and questioning your own patterns of thought and behaviour. Not in a critical way, but in a curious way – to deepen understanding.

But how can self-awareness become a habit?

Cultivate the practice of taking a step back and regarding yourself through other eyes – the eyes of a caring friend – and wonder openly about why you have acted in a certain way, and how it relates to other actions you've made.

The better you understand yourself, the easier it becomes to seek and recognise people and situations that align with you and your deepest wishes. And when you find yourself in situations that do not align – walk away.

DO THIS

1. Be curious about yourself and others.
2. Listen more than you speak.
3. Be compassionate with yourself. Understand that you are doing you best.
4. Set an intention to live in the here and how. Be present.
5. Spend quality time alone.
6. Start writing in a journal at the end of each day to become more aware of your own thoughts.

> 'Who looks outside, dreams; who looks inside, awakes.'
>
> CARL JUNG

26

RETURN TO YOUR CENTRE

5 MINUTES

Inside each of us is a place of peace. It's our core, our centre, where there is calm acceptance of everything. Do you know this place? And how much time do you spend there?

How often we return to our centre is a matter of habit. If you practice yoga or meditation you probably spend time there regularly. If not, put some time aside to go there intentionally. A daily 5-minute guided meditation or breathwork session is enough to strengthen your connection with inner peace. It might be something that you do in the morning before starting work, or as a way to recharge for the afternoon or mindfully wrap up the work day.

Once you get into the habit of spending time in this peaceful centre, it becomes easier to return quickly when you need to. A deep breath, closing your eyes or placing a hand on your heart can be a quick trigger to take you back to that nurturing core.

SD NR C

I am centred and grounded.

DO THIS

1. Diffuse grounding essential oils such as cedarwood, patchouli or clary sage.
2. Create a soothing soundscape by playing ambient music or binaural beats.
3. Chant om.

DID YOU KNOW?

The sacred Hindu chant 'om' – the sound of the Universe – actually has three syllables: A, U, M.

27

DAILY GRATITUDE HABIT

15 MINUTES

Gratitude is an emotional wonder-drug with proven benefits to mental, emotional and social health. It magnifies positive emotions, making us more optimistic, joyful and compassionate. Studies have even shown physical benefits like lower blood pressure and a stronger immune system.

Simply getting into the habit of thinking differently can free us from the negativity that stops us being as happy as we should be. Seeing our reality through gratitude-tinted glasses can change our perspective about ourselves, those around us and the lives we lead.

Starting a gratitude journal forces us to pay attention to the good things in life we might take for granted. Translating thoughts into concrete language makes us more aware, deepening the emotional impact.

Just before you go to sleep is a great time to journal your gratitude. You may even like to do it in bed, before you turn off the light. Spend your last few waking moments reflecting on the good things your day brought you, and then drift off into a contented sleep.

B EY NR

I am grateful for all that I have.

DO THIS

1. Devote a dedicated notebook to be your gratitude journal.
2. Keep the notebook by your bed to trigger the habit.
3. Write down three things that you are grateful for each day.
4. Go into detail about why you are grateful for each thing and how it makes you feel.
5. Take time to feel the strength of your gratitude, acknowledging each item on your list as a gift.
6. Every month (or when you need a lift), read over your journal entries.

> 'Once you begin to take note of the things you are grateful for, you begin to lose sight of the things that you lack.'

GERMANY KENT

28

SWEET SMELLING HABIT

5 MINUTES

We tend to overlook our sense of smell. We seek out beautiful scenes to look at, play music that pleases our ears, search out delicious tastes – but too often smell is left to fend for itself.

To get into the habit of feeding your olfactory pleasure centre, first tune into it: notice which smells grab your attention, which ones you love. Then introduce them into your environment. Start your day with an energising burst of rosemary or grapefruit, wind down in the evening with chamomile or lavender. Let your nose lead the way.

DO THIS

1. Put diffusers in rooms you use the most – where you work, where you relax – to remind you to diffuse oils.
2. Apply three drops to a cotton pad and breathe it in deeply 10 times.
3. Choose cleaning products with smells you like.

B NR

DID YOU KNOW?

People can detect at least one trillion distinct scents.

I am in touch with my senses.

29

GOOD TRANSITIONS HABIT

5 MINUTES

Our days are filled with transitions – between individual tasks and between larger blocks of time, like from work to personal time. We often naturally mark them with little rituals that signal to our brain it's time to switch gears, like a stretch or a cup of tea.

The workday commute acts as a kind of ritual, switching our state of mind between work-mode and home-mode. Even if you work from home, it's important to use ritual to give your brain time to reset and refocus – especially at the end of the workday when it can be hard to wind down, and the temptation can be to stay on a screen and simply change the browser window.

DO THIS

1. Tidy your desk and get it ready for starting tomorrow.
2. Write a quick to-do list for the next morning.
3. Change the music and lighting, switch the essential oil in the diffuser – modify your environment to reflect the change in focus.

S NR

I make the most of my time.

30

FIND PLEASURE IN CHORES

30 MINUTES

No one likes chores. But we all love the result – that contented little glow that only a sparkling tidy home can give you. So spring-clean your chore habit. Book in a regular time – 30 minutes should be enough if you do it weekly. (Saturday morning is the sweet spot.) Add bells and whistles so that it seems more like a joy than a drag. And bask in the glow of cleanliness.

DO THIS

1. Play your favourite music with the volume pumped up and sing along – loudly.
2. Listen to a podcast or audiobook you love.
3. Schedule cleaning time with your partner and enjoy doing it together.
4. Give yourself a reward afterwards.

RES

I take pride in keeping my home clean.

31

SCRAPE YOUR TONGUE

5 MINUTES

It removes bacteria, freshens your breath and makes food taste better. Flossing's neglected cousin, tongue-scraping is recommended by experts as part of everyday oral hygiene. It's an easy habit to get into – simply add it as an additional step after you brush and floss your teeth.

Oh, and use a scraper – they've been shown to remove 30 per cent more debris than a toothbrush.

DID YOU KNOW?

In Ayurveda, the tongue reflects the health of vital organs, including the heart, kidneys, liver, lungs, spleen and stomach.

RES NR

I care about my oral hygiene.

32
ONE BEAUTIFUL MOMENT

5 MINUTES

Those last moments before you go to bed are precious. As you close one day and prepare to take the long journey across dreams to the next, it's an opportunity to reflect, to decide what energy you want to take forward from this day.

Make it positive. Don't let yourself be transported by rumination or worries – this is the time to put the day's concerns behind you and meet your authentic, hopeful, optimistic self.

Take a few minutes to meditate or simply breathe. Feel your body, your presence in space and time. Simply be there and exist.

Confirm this habit by giving it concrete form in a journal. Note down one beautiful moment from your day. Anything from a flower you smelled to the kiss of a child – one simple, beautiful image to carry with you into sleep and beyond into your future.

B EY NR

I am a force of positive energy.

DO THIS

1. Diffuse a sweet, calming essential oil like lavender or ylang ylang.
2. Put your phone on its charging station, out of the bedroom.
3. Play calming, relaxing music.
4. Keep a journal at your beside as a trigger to write down your beautiful moment.

> 'Where we put our attention is where we live our lives.'
>
> SCOTT BARRY KAUFMAN

33

SLEEP SWEET SLEEP

30 MINUTES

Your bedtime ritual is one of your most important habits. It's all about sleep hygiene: a healthy routine that prepares you for bed, making a proper transition to the rejuvenating trip through the land of zeds.

Irregular pre-sleep habits are enough to cause insomnia, even if there aren't other factors, like stress or anxiety, at play. A regular bedtime ritual helps you wind down and de-stress, but also trains your brain to start to switch off in anticipation of reaching the pillow.

A bedtime ritual is a personal thing, and you'll tailor your own. It will include habits you already follow, like tooth-brushing and face-washing. Maybe you'll listen to soothing binaural beats as you follow your bathroom routine; maybe a short, relaxing series of stretches just before you climb into bed.

You might incorporate other habits you want to establish, like writing in a gratitude journal just before you turn the light out. Whatever you do, know that these habits are precious, and worth getting right.

SD NR

I am a good sleeper.

DO THIS

1. Make the hour or two before bed screen-free time.
2. Turn in early – the sleep you get before midnight is more restorative.
3. Write a brain-dump list of all you have to do the next day – then put it out of your mind.
4. Drink a cup of chamomile or valerian root herbal tea.
5. Spray your pillow with bergamot and lavender essential oils.
6. Do a full body scan or 5-minute meditation.

DID YOU KNOW?

We have four to six dreams every night, and forget 50% of them within 5 minutes of waking – and 90% within another 5 minutes.

34

BE OF SERVICE TO OTHERS

5 MINUTES

Giving is good for you. Acts of kindness and generosity make us feel more connected, and study after study shows that a feeling of social connectedness is vital for mental health and happiness. It gives us a sense of meaning in life, and the feeling that we are part of something bigger.

This is the idea behind the famous 'random act of kindness'. Compassionate, generous acts are like a virtuous circle, a ripple that spreads out from us. Yes, a kindness may well come back our way; but the reward is not in reciprocity. Kindness is its own reward – the act nourishes us, as much as it nourishes the receiver.

Set the intention to do something for another person every day – one small, kind thing – and the feel-good vibes you get will be enough to reinforce the habit.

B C G

I am a kind and caring person.

DO THIS

1. Run an errand for an elderly neighbour.
2. Hold the door open for someone.
3. Make a donation to a cause you care about.
4. Go through your clothes and donate them to a homeless shelter.
5. Pick up rubbish in a park or on the beach.
6. Make a batch of biscuits or cupcakes for a friend.
7. Pick a bunch of flowers from your garden and deliver them to a local old folks' home.
8. Donate cans of food from your cupboard to a local food bank.
9. Create care packs for people who are experiencing homelessness.
10. Box up your old clothes and send them to an upcycler.

> 'Look for a way to lift someone up. And if that's all you do, that's enough.'
>
> ELIZABETH LESSER

35

FIRE YOUR SYNAPSES

5 MINUTES

An easy dopamine hit, a bump for your short-term memory and a stress reliever – the real puzzle is, why aren't we doing more of them? Puzzles are a great way to shift your thinking, a perfect mini-ritual for when you want to transition from one activity to another. All that, and a brain-health bonus too. So get puzzling!

DO THIS

1. Do a crossword, sudoku, Wordle, or other puzzle with your morning coffee or tea.
2. Start learning a language lesson-by-lesson on Duolingo or Babbel.
3. Play Scrabble or Words with Friends on your phone.
4. Want more? Start a giant jigsaw puzzle – a fantastic mindful activity.

DID YOU KNOW?

The largest commercial jigsaw puzzle went on sale in 2011 and contained 32,256 pieces.

RES NR

I am mentally active and nimble.

36

STAY CONNECTED

5 MINUTES

Our connections to others are what keep us tethered to life. They nourish us and give us meaning. When we are down they keep us afloat and when we are up they're how we celebrate.

In the fog of the everyday, we can forget to keep these connections alive and humming. Set an intention to keep those you love close, and act on it regularly.

DO THIS

1. Call a friend or family member just for a chat.
2. Write thank-you notes.
3. Send a lovely text to a friend you haven't spoken to in a while.
4. Check in with an elderly neighbour.

> 'When you like a flower, you just pluck it. But when you love a flower, you water it daily.'
>
> ANONYMOUS

EY C G

I love and care for the people around me.

37

FIND THE SPACE BETWEEN YOUR THOUGHTS

5 MINUTES

Your thoughts are always there. Rushing, racing, searching for solutions to your tiniest questions and desires. It's one of life's deepest insights to realise – and fully accept – that you are not your thoughts. You are what is between them.

Meditation is a way of tapping into that authentic you. Practised over time, by teaching you to sit with discomfort and control your thoughts, it can help you respond to life's challenges from a more relaxed, mindful place. A daily 5-minute meditation might be the most life-changing habit you can start.

Progressive muscle relaxation is another way into the meditation space. It involves tensing then relaxing one body part at a time, allowing you to shift your focus from the mind's constant chatter to the simple messages of muscles and nerves.

Start small. Once a week, gradually build up your time until you can achieve a 20-minute meditation.

SD NR C

I am my authentic self.

DO THIS

1. Sit comfortably in a chair or lie down. Set a timer for 5 minutes.

2. Focus on your breath. Counting to five, slowly inhale starting with the belly, then the ribs, then the chest. Gently hold the breath for the fifth count.

3. Reverse this process to breathe out.

4. If thoughts enter your mind, observe them from a distance and gently let them go, returning your attention to your breath.

5. Visualise the tension leaving your body, escaping on your breath with every exhale.

> 'The thing about meditation is you become more and more you.'
>
> DAVID LYNCH

38

WALK

15 MINUTES

Our culture has a car habit, but that doesn't mean we have to adopt it. Before you get into the car, ask yourself – is this really necessary? Detach your car keys and keep them separate from your house keys to reinforce the question.

Once you drop the car habit, you'll feel benefits both physical and mental. Walking is a full-body exercise, with 200 muscles required to take just one step. It's low-impact, calming and addictive. Soon enough, you'll be looking for reasons to walk, and the further the better.

To turn up the dial, apply the principles of meditation to your walks. Tune in to your body and become aware of your posture and your gait. Then turn your awareness outwards, tuning into the sights, smells and sounds around you. Pay attention. Open your senses. Look for beauty, and when you find it, appreciate it with wonder and gratitude.

When your mind wanders off, come back to the rhythm of your stride and the sensation of your soles hitting the ground. Just walk.

M NR

I exercise my body whenever I have the chance.

DO THIS

1. Walk to the shops instead of taking the car.
2. Catch the train or tram from one station further along, and get off one station early.
3. If it's less than three floors, take the stairs.
4. Go for a 15-minute post-prandial walk after lunch or dinner.
5. Suggest to a friend you catch up over a long walk instead of a coffee.
6. Join a walking group.
7. Get a dog!

DID YOU KNOW?

If you take 9000 steps each day, in a lifetime that is 3.5 trips around the Earth.

39

CALM YOUR NERVOUS SYSTEM

10 MINUTES

When your sympathetic nervous system has been triggered, you know it. Rapid breathing, heavy heartbeats, jittering, changes in temperature – your body is preparing to fight or flee, even if all that happened was an uncomfortable meeting at work. It's stress central.

Recognising this state of stress is the first step. The second is having methods in place to calm the farm. You may need to try a few things, but once you know what works, you can get into the habit of taking that action when you feel yourself spiralling.

Stimulating the body's natural supply of oxytocin through touch and massage rapidly regulates the stress response. This feel-good neurotransmitter is the brain's foundation of trust and connection. The vagus nerve is your other fast-track to peace – activate it by massage or using your vocal chords.

Whatever your technique, know that you have it in your toolkit, ready to pull out next time the jitters hit.

SD RES NR

I know how to soothe myself when I feel out of sorts.

DO THIS

1. Place your hand on your heart and breathe deeply in and out five times.
2. Give yourself a foot massage by rotating your ankle, rubbing your sole in short strokes and gently stretching your toes back and forth.
3. Massage warm almond oil into your skin and the crown of your head.
4. Submerge: float in a body of water or take a long, hot bath.
5. Share a 20-second, full-body hug with a willing partner.
6. Massage your vagus nerve – gently rub the back of your head, where the top of your neck nestles into the skull.
7. Do some doodling or colouring in.
8. Chant, hum or sing to yourself.
9. Practice self-compassion: remind yourself it's OK to feel freaked out and you haven't done anything 'wrong'.

'You are the sky. Everything else – it's just the weather.'

PEMA CHÖDRÖN

40

TEND TO SOMETHING

5 MINUTES

B RES NR

I have a green thumb.

The research is in: gardening is good for you. A growing list of studies backs the idea that gardening benefits both mental and physical health. Makes sense. It's a natural mindfulness exercise, a little link to nature, a daily interaction with beauty.

Place your plant somewhere you'll see it every day. Make watering it part of your weekly cleaning ritual, and get into the habit of checking in every day to make sure it's doing OK, maybe as part of your morning routine.

Give it a name. You may even want to chat to it from time to time.

DO THIS

1. Start with a succulent or easy-care indoor plant.
2. Plant a pot of herbs near your kitchen window.
3. No backyard? Join a shared garden.

DID YOU KNOW?

Plants are thought to reduce levels of cortisol, the stress hormone.

41

ACCEPT WHAT IS

5 MINUTES

It's called the Golden Rule, and it goes something like this: 'Treat others as you would like others to treat you.' But somehow, we often treat ourselves with *less* kindness and compassion than we show to others. We don't expect our friends to be perfect, so why do we set such high standards for ourselves? Self-acceptance means embracing all that we are, strengths and weaknesses. It's the habit that corresponds most closely with life satisfaction, so it's an important one to start practicing.

DO THIS

1. Speak to yourself with kindness.
2. Compare yourself only to your past self, not to others.
3. Forgive yourself for mistakes – acknowledge them and move on.
4. Repeat affirmations for self-love every day.

'I woke up like this. Flawless.'

BEYONCÉ

RES NR

I love myself as I am.

42

INTEGRATE EXERCISE

5 MINUTES

When it comes to starting an exercise habit, we struggle with two hurdles (and that's not running-track hurdles): motivation and time. The motivation hurdle is that little voice in our head, piping up with variations on, 'But I can't be *bothered*!' The trick is to fool it – and confound the time hurdle as well – by starting your exercise practice with a habit so insignificant that your lazy inner voice will barely notice it.

Going to the gym every day involves a lot of friction. Getting ready, getting yourself there, the time commitment – there are many hurdles to clear, all of them opportunities for demotivation. So start with something seamless. Something you can do by simply stepping out your front door, like going for a run. Or something you can do at home, like bodyweight exercises (squats, push-ups, sit-ups).

Commit to five minutes, every day. If it's too hard to start with, just put on your running shoes and go for a five-minute walk. Anything that gets you primed and out the door. Simply get in the habit of using that time for 'running'. Let the actual running come later.

M

I have a fit, healthy body.

DO THIS

1. Exercise while listening to your favourite music or podcast – it's a built-in reward.

2. Do your exercise at the same time every day – piggy-back it off a regular event such as getting home from work.

3. Be kind to yourself – habits take time.

4. Time your exercise so that it's followed by something you enjoy, or give yourself a little reward after it.

5. Join a running or walking group to reinforce your habit, or do it with a friend.

> 'A habit cannot be tossed out the window; it must be coaxed down the stairs a step at a time.'
>
> MARK TWAIN

43

HEALTHY RELATIONSHIP HABIT

1 HOUR

EY NR C

We have a happy, loving relationship.

Love is magic. But also, it's not. Successful relationships succeed less thanks to romantic fairydust than to couples building and maintaining healthy habits. 'Habitual' might sound boring, but it's the opposite – it's the lifeblood of long-term love.

Especially when you live with your partner, happy habits help the wheels of cohabitation turn smoothly. You will fall into habits whether intentional or not – some will be good, and some may not be. Do a quick audit of your couple habits – give the positive ones a tick, but pay special attention to the negative ones. Are there habits you need to change?

Communication habits are the most important. Make sure you're building habits that provide space to connect authentically and honestly. You might decide on a weekly check-in – in a specific place, at a specific time – that's dedicated to a debrief of 'the week that was' in your relationship. Discuss anything that's come up, air what needs to be aired, talk through any bumps. A regular habit like this will keep the lines of communication open and prevent any unspoken irks to fester and grow.

DO THIS

1. Connect emotionally every day.
2. Don't make assumptions about your partner's feelings – ask them.
3. Say sorry and mean it.
4. Find little ways to show how much you appreciate them.
5. Do chores together.
6. Balance 'me time' and 'we time'.
7. Eat at least one meal together every day – no screens.
8. Exercise together.
9. Say goodbye (and hello) properly.
10. Leave notes for each other.

> 'See the light in each other. Be the light for each other.'
>
> ANONYMOUS

44

MAKE TIME TO LET GO

10 MINUTES

Unintentionally, we can form a habit of holding on to things that aren't good for us. The past, painful thoughts or memories, unhealthy relationships. Becoming aware of the things that we welcome into our lives that we can't control and that don't serve us is the first step to flipping this habit.

Make a list of the things in your life that worry you or get you down. Identify the things that you can't control and the things you can. The things you can control are things to work on – take the first step by starting to create a micro-habit around them.

For the things you can't control, it's time to let them go. Remember that the only power these things have over you is the way you think about them. Don't worry what others think about you – you are the only critic that counts. Switch your habitual thinking to loosen your grasp on the unhelpful things in your life.

NR

I am free.

DO THIS

1. Understand that your reality might not be exactly what you had planned, and that's OK.
2. Accept that you can't control anyone else's actions – only your own.
3. Stop blaming others – accept responsibility for your own life and choices.
4. Allow yourself to make mistakes, and forgive yourself easily.
5. Surround yourself with people who love and support you.
6. Spend time doing things that bring you joy.

> 'Letting go isn't a one-time thing, it's something you have to do every day, over and over again.'
>
> DAWSON'S CREEK

45

LISTEN

10 MINUTES

A sound bath is a kind of meditation that uses waves of sound to incite peace and healing. It calls on instruments like gongs, singing bowls, percussion, chimes, rattles, tuning forks and even the human voice. But you don't need to find a sound therapy practitioner to tap into the healing power of sound. Get into the habit of attuning your ears to the soothing soundscapes all around.

DO THIS

1. Search 'sound bath' on Spotify or YouTube for some DIY sound therapy.
2. Look up binaural beats or solfeggio frequencies to open your ears to the sound of the cosmos.
3. Tune in to the birds in the trees and wind in the branches.

DID YOU KNOW?

Your ears never sleep. They continue to collect all the sounds around you.

SD NR

I am in tune with the world around me.

46

MOVE SOFTLY, SPEAK SLOWLY

1 MINUTE

Do you find yourself rushing around and you don't know why? Do you trip over your own tongue or, maybe worse, trip over your own feet? We can find ourselves in a whirlwind of activity that's self-perpetuating. There's busy because you have a lot to do, and then there's busy just because you're in the habit of always being busy.

Instead, stop and whisper to yourself simply 'slow down'. It's a reminder that there is no external force insisting that you hurry up. It's just you – and you have the power to turn down the volume.

'Nature does not hurry, yet everything is accomplished.'

LAO TZU

SD

I am gentle and considered.

47

CREATE, BUILD, MAKE, DO

30 MINUTES

Creative hobbies are so established as a balm for mental health that they're often given as medical advice.

Getting creative is like cross-training for your brain. For those of us who aren't professional artists, arty hobbies allow us to give our brain's right hemisphere a workout – that's the side that handles creative thinking. New brain cells grow and new neural connections are made. The practical upshot: our brains are more supple, our solutions more creative. We are literally more well-rounded (our brains are, anyway).

Plus, engaging in mindful activity puts us into a flow state that releases stress and lowers cortisol levels.

So pick up a guitar or a paintbrush, buy a colouring book, learn to macramé, dust off the sewing machine, ask your granny to teach you to crochet, take a bookbinding course, throw a lump of clay on a pottery wheel, or make funny animals out of fruit and vegetables. Whatever creative activity you make your new habit, it's going to be good for your brain, and your soul.

B EY NR

I have interesting hobbies.

DO THIS

1. Choose something you've always been interested in, or you remember enjoying as a child.
2. Start small – commit to 30 minutes a week.
3. Buy just what you need – crayons, a few paints, a little wool – and keep it somewhere you can see it as a cue.
4. If you can, dedicate a space to it.
5. Google for online courses, find your tribe on Instagram or TikTok – get inspiration wherever you can.
6. If it's going well, consider taking a course to reinforce the habit and boost your skills.
7. Join a group of fellow crafters – your habit will become more concrete when it's part of a social activity.

DID YOU KNOW?

Studies have found that people with hobbies continue to be happier and experience lower levels of depression and negativity for up to a full day after practice ends.

48

SIFT YOUR MIND

5 MINUTES

SIFTing is a process that helps us quickly connect with how we're feeling. You could use it as an everyday self-check-in habit, or a ritual to turn to when you feel scattered and in need of emotional grounding. The more you use it, the more self-aware and in touch with your inner life you'll be.

Find a quiet place to sit, close your eyes and follow the four steps. Afterwards acknowledge and accept what you experienced, without judgement – whatever comes up for you is what comes up for you.

DO THIS

1. Senses: Think about what you are sensing physically with your body.
2. Images: What appears in your mind's eye?
3. Feelings: How are you feeling? Try to put a name to the feelings, or just be aware of your emotional state.
4. Thoughts: Where are your thoughts?

SD C

I am in touch with my inner self.

49

ACUPRESSURE MAT

15 MINUTES

RB NR

I know how to regulate my energy levels.

The mid-afternoon slump is real. It's thanks to your circadian rhythm (aka internal body clock), which is responsible for waking you in the morning and making you drowsy at night. It takes a natural dip between 2 pm and 4 pm, explaining your sudden need for coffee or chocolate.

Drop that habit by giving yourself an energy boost (and reduce stress, relieve muscle tension and ease pain) with a simple 15-minute lie-down – if you lie down on an acupressure mat. Like a yoga mat with a bed-of-nails twist, acupressure mats mimic the effects of acupuncture in stimulating the body's pressure points to help the flow of *chi*, or energy.

If that doesn't appeal, go for a quick walk around the block or do a stretching session. And if you can, a quick nap might be just what your circadian rhythm needs to make it through until bedtime.

DID YOU KNOW?

The optimal length of time for a nap is 26 minutes.

50
CELEBRATE OTHERS

5 MINUTES

Being truly happy for someone else is precious – after all, it involves being happy. Emotions are contagious and self-replicating. When you enjoy the success of others, you start a feedback loop of positive thinking in your own mind – and it works even if you have to fake your enthusiasm at first.

Comparison is the thief of joy. Don't be tempted by the snarky little voice that wants you to feel jealous or ask why *you* didn't get that raise or marriage proposal. Instead, use your friends' and colleagues' achievements as inspiration and learning, while allowing yourself to feel uncomplicatedly happy for their good news.

When you're putting the spotlight on someone else, you're not focusing solely on yourself. It's a form of positive empathy, wearing the happy shoes of someone who's experiencing joy. It's a form of giving that strengthens your connection with that person. And it's good for the soul.

C G

I make other people feel good about themselves.

DO THIS

1. Be authentic when you congratulate someone – be truly happy for them.
2. Organise events to celebrate successes and milestones.
3. Use the good news of others as a trigger for gratitude for what you have yourself.
4. Remember birthdays and other special days, and mark them with a card, a note or a call.
5. Don't allow the moment to disappear – remember the achievement and bring it up in future conversations.

'Appreciation is a wonderful thing. It makes what is excellent in others belong to us as well.'

VOLTAIRE

SECTION THREE

Reflections

How did you go?

FEEDBACK IS YOUR FRIEND

Give yourself the gift of feedback by tracking your efforts to adopt new habits. The better you track and reflect on your efforts, the more you learn and grow, and the closer to your goals you will be.

HABIT-BY-HABIT

In this section of the book, you will find a page dedicated to each habit, providing you with the opportunity to reflect on how a habit worked (or didn't work) for you. Right at the end of this section, there is further space for you to ponder some bigger questions about the impact of your new-found habits on your life.

WHAT, WHEN, WHY

When reflecting on individual habits, first make a quick note of the 'what, when and why'. 'What' is your version of the habit – what you actually did. 'When' is the time and frequency with which you did it. And 'why', of course, is what motivated you to pick that habit and experiment with it.

NEXT STEPS

Perhaps you have found some habits helpful, others a bit ho-hum and yet others no good at all for you. There is a lot to be learned from these reactions. Use the questions on each habit spread to help you explore this. If a habit worked for you, then you will want to stay the course. How will you do that? Stretch your mind to think of achievable ways to stay committed to success. If a habit didn't resonate, that could present an opportunity to rethink it. Are there ways it could be modified to improve its usefulness to you? Ensure you give adequate thought to this possibility and you may be able to design another awesome habit to add to your toolkit. If a habit definitely didn't work for you, then don't dismiss the learnings. There is probably a good reason why. Maybe you are already winning in that area and didn't really need it. That's a tick for you! Or maybe you are already doing enough – another great learning. Use the space provided in this book to reflect on these questions and hold yourself accountable for the ups and downs of your journey to a less stressful life.

> 'It's on the strength of observation and reflection that one finds a way. So we must dig and delve unceasingly.'
>
> CLAUDE MONET

01 MORNING PAGES

WHAT I DID

WHEN I DID IT

WHY I DID IT

If this habit worked for you, why do you think that is, and how will you stay committed?
Can you modify or improve on it? If it didn't work for you, why do you think that is?

I TRIED THIS ☐ **I LIKE THIS** ☐ **THIS DID NOT WORK FOR ME** ☐

02 SET YOUR ALARM

WHAT I DID

WHEN I DID IT

WHY I DID IT

If this habit worked for you, why do you think that is, and how will you stay committed? Can you modify or improve on it? If it didn't work for you, why do you think that is?

I TRIED THIS ☐ **I LIKE THIS** ☐ **THIS DID NOT WORK FOR ME** ☐

03 STRETCH

WHAT I DID

WHEN I DID IT

WHY I DID IT

If this habit worked for you, why do you think that is, and how will you stay committed? Can you modify or improve on it? If it didn't work for you, why do you think that is?

I TRIED THIS ☐ **I LIKE THIS** ☐ **THIS DID NOT WORK FOR ME** ☐

04 COOL AND CLEANSE

WHAT I DID

WHEN I DID IT

WHY I DID IT

If this habit worked for you, why do you think that is, and how will you stay committed? Can you modify or improve on it? If it didn't work for you, why do you think that is?

I TRIED THIS ☐ **I LIKE THIS** ☐ **THIS DID NOT WORK FOR ME** ☐

05 SAY GOODBYE WITH CARE

WHAT I DID

WHEN I DID IT

WHY I DID IT

If this habit worked for you, why do you think that is, and how will you stay committed? Can you modify or improve on it? If it didn't work for you, why do you think that is?

I TRIED THIS ☐ **I LIKE THIS** ☐ **THIS DID NOT WORK FOR ME** ☐

06 MAKE YOUR BED

WHAT I DID ______

WHEN I DID IT ______

WHY I DID IT ______

If this habit worked for you, why do you think that is, and how will you stay committed? Can you modify or improve on it? If it didn't work for you, why do you think that is?

I TRIED THIS ☐ **I LIKE THIS** ☐ **THIS DID NOT WORK FOR ME** ☐

07 LEAVE THE HOUSE MINDFULLY

WHAT I DID

WHEN I DID IT

WHY I DID IT

If this habit worked for you, why do you think that is, and how will you stay committed? Can you modify or improve on it? If it didn't work for you, why do you think that is?

I TRIED THIS ☐ **I LIKE THIS** ☐ **THIS DID NOT WORK FOR ME** ☐

08 FOCUS ON THE BREATH

WHAT I DID ______________________________

WHEN I DID IT ______________________________

WHY I DID IT ______________________________

If this habit worked for you, why do you think that is, and how will you stay committed? Can you modify or improve on it? If it didn't work for you, why do you think that is?

I TRIED THIS ☐ **I LIKE THIS** ☐ **THIS DID NOT WORK FOR ME** ☐

09 TECH CONTROL HABIT

WHAT I DID

WHEN I DID IT

WHY I DID IT

If this habit worked for you, why do you think that is, and how will you stay committed? Can you modify or improve on it? If it didn't work for you, why do you think that is?

I TRIED THIS ☐ **I LIKE THIS** ☐ **THIS DID NOT WORK FOR ME** ☐

10 DO THE LIFE ADMIN

WHAT I DID

WHEN I DID IT

WHY I DID IT

If this habit worked for you, why do you think that is, and how will you stay committed? Can you modify or improve on it? If it didn't work for you, why do you think that is?

I TRIED THIS ☐ I LIKE THIS ☐ THIS DID NOT WORK FOR ME ☐

11 BODY SCAN

WHAT I DID

WHEN I DID IT

WHY I DID IT

If this habit worked for you, why do you think that is, and how will you stay committed? Can you modify or improve on it? If it didn't work for you, why do you think that is?

I TRIED THIS ☐ **I LIKE THIS** ☐ **THIS DID NOT WORK FOR ME** ☐

12 TAP INTO FEELINGS OF DISCOMFORT

WHAT I DID

WHEN I DID IT

WHY I DID IT

If this habit worked for you, why do you think that is, and how will you stay committed?
Can you modify or improve on it? If it didn't work for you, why do you think that is?

I TRIED THIS ☐ **I LIKE THIS** ☐ **THIS DID NOT WORK FOR ME** ☐

13 EAT MINDFULLY

WHAT I DID

WHEN I DID IT

WHY I DID IT

If this habit worked for you, why do you think that is, and how will you stay committed? Can you modify or improve on it? If it didn't work for you, why do you think that is?

I TRIED THIS ☐ **I LIKE THIS** ☐ **THIS DID NOT WORK FOR ME** ☐

14 BE PRESENT WITH OTHERS

WHAT I DID

WHEN I DID IT

WHY I DID IT

If this habit worked for you, why do you think that is, and how will you stay committed? Can you modify or improve on it? If it didn't work for you, why do you think that is?

I TRIED THIS ☐ **I LIKE THIS** ☐ **THIS DID NOT WORK FOR ME** ☐

15 STAY REGULATED

WHAT I DID

WHEN I DID IT

WHY I DID IT

If this habit worked for you, why do you think that is, and how will you stay committed? Can you modify or improve on it? If it didn't work for you, why do you think that is?

I TRIED THIS ☐ **I LIKE THIS** ☐ **THIS DID NOT WORK FOR ME** ☐

16 SAY NO

WHAT I DID ______________________________

WHEN I DID IT ______________________________

WHY I DID IT ______________________________

If this habit worked for you, why do you think that is, and how will you stay committed? Can you modify or improve on it? If it didn't work for you, why do you think that is?

I TRIED THIS ☐ **I LIKE THIS** ☐ **THIS DID NOT WORK FOR ME** ☐

17 REHYDRATE

WHAT I DID

WHEN I DID IT

WHY I DID IT

If this habit worked for you, why do you think that is, and how will you stay committed? Can you modify or improve on it? If it didn't work for you, why do you think that is?

I TRIED THIS ☐ **I LIKE THIS** ☐ **THIS DID NOT WORK FOR ME** ☐

18 MAKE TIME TO BE OUTSIDE

WHAT I DID ____________________

WHEN I DID IT ____________________

WHY I DID IT ____________________

If this habit worked for you, why do you think that is, and how will you stay committed? Can you modify or improve on it? If it didn't work for you, why do you think that is?

I TRIED THIS ☐ **I LIKE THIS** ☐ **THIS DID NOT WORK FOR ME** ☐

19 CONNECT WITH SPIRIT

WHAT I DID

WHEN I DID IT

WHY I DID IT

If this habit worked for you, why do you think that is, and how will you stay committed? Can you modify or improve on it? If it didn't work for you, why do you think that is?

I TRIED THIS ☐ **I LIKE THIS** ☐ **THIS DID NOT WORK FOR ME** ☐

20 TAKE NO SIDES

WHAT I DID

WHEN I DID IT

WHY I DID IT

If this habit worked for you, why do you think that is, and how will you stay committed? Can you modify or improve on it? If it didn't work for you, why do you think that is?

I TRIED THIS ☐ I LIKE THIS ☐ THIS DID NOT WORK FOR ME ☐

21 SWAY AWAY

WHAT I DID

WHEN I DID IT

WHY I DID IT

If this habit worked for you, why do you think that is, and how will you stay committed? Can you modify or improve on it? If it didn't work for you, why do you think that is?

I TRIED THIS ☐ **I LIKE THIS** ☐ **THIS DID NOT WORK FOR ME** ☐

22 FIND DAILY JOY

WHAT I DID

WHEN I DID IT

WHY I DID IT

If this habit worked for you, why do you think that is, and how will you stay committed?
Can you modify or improve on it? If it didn't work for you, why do you think that is?

I TRIED THIS ☐ I LIKE THIS ☐ THIS DID NOT WORK FOR ME ☐

23 YOUR HEALTHY HOME HABITS

WHAT I DID

WHEN I DID IT

WHY I DID IT

If this habit worked for you, why do you think that is, and how will you stay committed? Can you modify or improve on it? If it didn't work for you, why do you think that is?

I TRIED THIS ☐ **I LIKE THIS** ☐ **THIS DID NOT WORK FOR ME** ☐

24 POWER OF PAUSE

WHAT I DID ____________________

WHEN I DID IT ____________________

WHY I DID IT ____________________

If this habit worked for you, why do you think that is, and how will you stay committed? Can you modify or improve on it? If it didn't work for you, why do you think that is?

I TRIED THIS ☐ **I LIKE THIS** ☐ **THIS DID NOT WORK FOR ME** ☐

25 PRACTISE SELF-AWARENESS

WHAT I DID

WHEN I DID IT

WHY I DID IT

If this habit worked for you, why do you think that is, and how will you stay committed? Can you modify or improve on it? If it didn't work for you, why do you think that is?

I TRIED THIS ☐ **I LIKE THIS** ☐ **THIS DID NOT WORK FOR ME** ☐

26 RETURN TO YOUR CENTRE

WHAT I DID

WHEN I DID IT

WHY I DID IT

If this habit worked for you, why do you think that is, and how will you stay committed?
Can you modify or improve on it? If it didn't work for you, why do you think that is?

I TRIED THIS ☐ **I LIKE THIS** ☐ **THIS DID NOT WORK FOR ME** ☐

27 DAILY GRATITUDE HABIT

WHAT I DID

WHEN I DID IT

WHY I DID IT

If this habit worked for you, why do you think that is, and how will you stay committed? Can you modify or improve on it? If it didn't work for you, why do you think that is?

I TRIED THIS ☐ **I LIKE THIS** ☐ **THIS DID NOT WORK FOR ME** ☐

28 SWEET SMELLING HABIT

WHAT I DID

WHEN I DID IT

WHY I DID IT

If this habit worked for you, why do you think that is, and how will you stay committed? Can you modify or improve on it? If it didn't work for you, why do you think that is?

I TRIED THIS ☐ **I LIKE THIS** ☐ **THIS DID NOT WORK FOR ME** ☐

29 GOOD TRANSITIONS HABIT

WHAT I DID

WHEN I DID IT

WHY I DID IT

If this habit worked for you, why do you think that is, and how will you stay committed?
Can you modify or improve on it? If it didn't work for you, why do you think that is?

I TRIED THIS ☐ **I LIKE THIS** ☐ **THIS DID NOT WORK FOR ME** ☐

30 FIND PLEASURE IN CHORES

WHAT I DID

WHEN I DID IT

WHY I DID IT

If this habit worked for you, why do you think that is, and how will you stay committed? Can you modify or improve on it? If it didn't work for you, why do you think that is?

I TRIED THIS ☐ I LIKE THIS ☐ THIS DID NOT WORK FOR ME ☐

31 SCRAPE YOUR TONGUE

WHAT I DID

WHEN I DID IT

WHY I DID IT

If this habit worked for you, why do you think that is, and how will you stay committed? Can you modify or improve on it? If it didn't work for you, why do you think that is?

I TRIED THIS ☐ I LIKE THIS ☐ THIS DID NOT WORK FOR ME ☐

32 ONE BEAUTIFUL MOMENT

WHAT I DID

WHEN I DID IT

WHY I DID IT

If this habit worked for you, why do you think that is, and how will you stay committed? Can you modify or improve on it? If it didn't work for you, why do you think that is?

I TRIED THIS ☐ **I LIKE THIS** ☐ **THIS DID NOT WORK FOR ME** ☐

33 SLEEP SWEET SLEEP

WHAT I DID

WHEN I DID IT

WHY I DID IT

If this habit worked for you, why do you think that is, and how will you stay committed? Can you modify or improve on it? If it didn't work for you, why do you think that is?

I TRIED THIS ☐ **I LIKE THIS** ☐ **THIS DID NOT WORK FOR ME** ☐

34 BE OF SERVICE TO OTHERS

WHAT I DID

WHEN I DID IT

WHY I DID IT

If this habit worked for you, why do you think that is, and how will you stay committed? Can you modify or improve on it? If it didn't work for you, why do you think that is?

I TRIED THIS ☐ **I LIKE THIS** ☐ **THIS DID NOT WORK FOR ME** ☐

35 FIRE YOUR SYNAPSES

WHAT I DID

WHEN I DID IT

WHY I DID IT

If this habit worked for you, why do you think that is, and how will you stay committed? Can you modify or improve on it? If it didn't work for you, why do you think that is?

I TRIED THIS ☐ I LIKE THIS ☐ THIS DID NOT WORK FOR ME ☐

36 STAY CONNECTED

WHAT I DID ____________________

WHEN I DID IT ____________________

WHY I DID IT ____________________

If this habit worked for you, why do you think that is, and how will you stay committed? Can you modify or improve on it? If it didn't work for you, why do you think that is?

I TRIED THIS ☐ **I LIKE THIS** ☐ **THIS DID NOT WORK FOR ME** ☐

37 FIND THE SPACE BETWEEN YOUR THOUGHTS

WHAT I DID

WHEN I DID IT

WHY I DID IT

If this habit worked for you, why do you think that is, and how will you stay committed? Can you modify or improve on it? If it didn't work for you, why do you think that is?

I TRIED THIS ☐ **I LIKE THIS** ☐ **THIS DID NOT WORK FOR ME** ☐

38 WALK

WHAT I DID

WHEN I DID IT

WHY I DID IT

If this habit worked for you, why do you think that is, and how will you stay committed? Can you modify or improve on it? If it didn't work for you, why do you think that is?

I TRIED THIS ☐ I LIKE THIS ☐ THIS DID NOT WORK FOR ME ☐

39 CALM YOUR NERVOUS SYSTEM

WHAT I DID

WHEN I DID IT

WHY I DID IT

If this habit worked for you, why do you think that is, and how will you stay committed? Can you modify or improve on it? If it didn't work for you, why do you think that is?

I TRIED THIS ☐ **I LIKE THIS** ☐ **THIS DID NOT WORK FOR ME** ☐

40 TEND TO SOMETHING

WHAT I DID

WHEN I DID IT

WHY I DID IT

If this habit worked for you, why do you think that is, and how will you stay committed?
Can you modify or improve on it? If it didn't work for you, why do you think that is?

I TRIED THIS ☐ **I LIKE THIS** ☐ **THIS DID NOT WORK FOR ME** ☐

41 ACCEPT WHAT IS

WHAT I DID

WHEN I DID IT

WHY I DID IT

If this habit worked for you, why do you think that is, and how will you stay committed? Can you modify or improve on it? If it didn't work for you, why do you think that is?

I TRIED THIS ☐ **I LIKE THIS** ☐ **THIS DID NOT WORK FOR ME** ☐

42 INTEGRATE EXERCISE

WHAT I DID

WHEN I DID IT

WHY I DID IT

If this habit worked for you, why do you think that is, and how will you stay committed? Can you modify or improve on it? If it didn't work for you, why do you think that is?

I TRIED THIS ☐ **I LIKE THIS** ☐ **THIS DID NOT WORK FOR ME** ☐

43 HEALTHY RELATIONSHIP HABIT

WHAT I DID

WHEN I DID IT

WHY I DID IT

If this habit worked for you, why do you think that is, and how will you stay committed? Can you modify or improve on it? If it didn't work for you, why do you think that is?

I TRIED THIS ☐ I LIKE THIS ☐ THIS DID NOT WORK FOR ME ☐

44 MAKE TIME TO LET GO

WHAT I DID

WHEN I DID IT

WHY I DID IT

If this habit worked for you, why do you think that is, and how will you stay committed? Can you modify or improve on it? If it didn't work for you, why do you think that is?

I TRIED THIS ☐ I LIKE THIS ☐ THIS DID NOT WORK FOR ME ☐

45 LISTEN

WHAT I DID

WHEN I DID IT

WHY I DID IT

If this habit worked for you, why do you think that is, and how will you stay committed? Can you modify or improve on it? If it didn't work for you, why do you think that is?

I TRIED THIS ☐ I LIKE THIS ☐ THIS DID NOT WORK FOR ME ☐

46 MOVE SOFTLY, SPEAK SLOWLY

WHAT I DID

WHEN I DID IT

WHY I DID IT

If this habit worked for you, why do you think that is, and how will you stay committed?
Can you modify or improve on it? If it didn't work for you, why do you think that is?

I TRIED THIS ☐ **I LIKE THIS** ☐ **THIS DID NOT WORK FOR ME** ☐

47 CREATE, BUILD, MAKE, DO

WHAT I DID

WHEN I DID IT

WHY I DID IT

If this habit worked for you, why do you think that is, and how will you stay committed? Can you modify or improve on it? If it didn't work for you, why do you think that is?

I TRIED THIS ☐ **I LIKE THIS** ☐ **THIS DID NOT WORK FOR ME** ☐

48 SIFT YOUR MIND

WHAT I DID

WHEN I DID IT

WHY I DID IT

If this habit worked for you, why do you think that is, and how will you stay committed? Can you modify or improve on it? If it didn't work for you, why do you think that is?

I TRIED THIS ☐ I LIKE THIS ☐ THIS DID NOT WORK FOR ME ☐

49 ACUPRESSURE MAT

WHAT I DID

WHEN I DID IT

WHY I DID IT

If this habit worked for you, why do you think that is, and how will you stay committed? Can you modify or improve on it? If it didn't work for you, why do you think that is?

I TRIED THIS ☐ **I LIKE THIS** ☐ **THIS DID NOT WORK FOR ME** ☐

50 CELEBRATE OTHERS

WHAT I DID

WHEN I DID IT

WHY I DID IT

If this habit worked for you, why do you think that is, and how will you stay committed? Can you modify or improve on it? If it didn't work for you, why do you think that is?

I TRIED THIS ☐ **I LIKE THIS** ☐ **THIS DID NOT WORK FOR ME** ☐

Which habits 'stuck' and made the biggest impact on you, and why do you think that is?

How are you doing in terms of your goal for less stress in your life, and what role have your new habits had in helping you achieve this goal?

In what ways have your new habits helped you feel differently about yourself, your relationship to others and your life generally?

What has been the best outcome (or outcomes) for you of following the ideas in this book?

Thinking about a successful new habit, what did you learn that you might be able to apply to future habits you'd like to embrace?

HERRON

First Published in 2023 by Herron Book Distributors Pty Ltd
14 Manton St
Morningside
QLD 4170
www.herronbooks.com

Captain Honey

Custom book production by Captain Honey Pty Ltd
12 Station Street
Bangalow
NSW 2479
www.captainhoney.com.au

Cataloguing-in-Publication. A catalogue record for this book is available from the National Library of Australia

ISBN 978-1-922944-46-7

Printed and bound in China